# Whole Body Reset Diet Cookbook 2024

Revitalize Your Life Through Mindful Eating
and Wholesome Ingredients

**Ennis James**

# Table of Contents

# Introduction

In the heart of downtown, amidst the aroma of freshly brewed coffee and the hum of city life, Emma found herself at a crossroads. Her hectic schedule as a marketing executive left little time for self-care, and her energy levels were plummeting. It was then that she stumbled upon a vibrant bookstore, its windows adorned with enticing displays of health and wellness.

Stepping inside, Emma's eyes fell upon a book that seemed to shimmer with promise: Whole Body Reset Diet Cookbook 2024. The cover, adorned with vibrant images of wholesome meals and energized faces, beckoned her closer. Intrigued, she flipped open the pages.

Within its crisp, inviting pages, Emma discovered a treasure trove of more than just recipes. The cookbook unfolded a comprehensive guide to revitalizing her entire being. Each recipe was carefully crafted to nourish not just the body, but the soul—a perfect harmony of flavors and nutrients designed to restore vitality and balance.

As Emma delved deeper, she found herself captivated by the cookbook's approach. It wasn't just about shedding pounds; it was about embracing a lifestyle that radiated wellness from within. The introduction illuminated the principles of the Whole Body Reset Diet—simple yet profound strategies to cleanse, rejuvenate, and sustain.

The breakfast section offered a symphony of flavors, from antioxidant-rich smoothie bowls to hearty quinoa porridge, promising to kick-start her mornings with sustained energy. Lunchtime beckoned with vibrant salads, nourishing wraps, and comforting soups—perfect for fueling her through busy afternoons without the dreaded midday slump.

Dinner became a celebration of wholesome indulgence. Emma envisioned herself savoring dishes like grilled salmon with asparagus, or perhaps indulging in a cozy bowl of lentil soup with fresh herbs. Each recipe was a testament to the cookbook's commitment to flavor, nutrition, and simplicity— a true culinary journey towards vitality.

But it wasn't just about the meals. Whole Body Reset Diet Cookbook 2024 offered practical meal plans tailored to different wellness goals, whether it was weight loss, muscle building, or simply maintaining a balanced lifestyle. Emma could see herself effortlessly navigating her weekly meals with newfound confidence and creativity.

As she read on, Emma felt a sense of empowerment. This wasn't just another cookbook; it was a roadmap to reclaiming her health and vitality. The cookbook's thoughtful insights, backed by nutritional expertise, assured her that every recipe was a step towards a brighter, more energized future.

With a smile of determination, Emma decided to bring the Whole Body Reset Diet Cookbook 2024 home. It wasn't just a purchase—it was an investment in herself, a commitment to prioritize her well-being amidst life's demands. She knew that with each recipe she tried, she would be nurturing not just her body, but her spirit—a journey of wellness that would resonate far beyond her kitchen.

And so, armed with her newfound treasure, Emma embarked on a journey of transformation. With every delicious bite and every revitalizing meal, she was reminded that true wellness begins from within—and that the Whole Body Reset Diet Cookbook 2024 was her trusted companion on this empowering path.

---

This story aims to illustrate the transformative power and holistic approach of the Whole Body Reset Diet Cookbook 2024, enticing potential buyers with its promise of vitality, flavor, and sustainable wellness.

# What is the Whole Body Reset Diet?

The Whole Body Reset Diet, as outlined in the Whole Body Reset Diet Cookbook 2024, represents a holistic approach to revitalizing one's health and well-being. At its core, this dietary plan goes beyond mere weight loss goals, focusing instead on resetting the body's systems to achieve optimal functioning. It acknowledges that modern lifestyles often lead to nutrient imbalances, inflammation, and sluggish metabolism, which can impact overall vitality and energy levels. By following this diet, individuals aim to restore balance and vitality through nutrient-dense foods that support cellular health and overall wellness.

Central to the Whole Body Reset Diet is the emphasis on whole, unprocessed foods. The cookbook encourages the consumption of fresh fruits and vegetables, lean proteins, whole grains, and healthy fats. These foods are not only rich in essential nutrients but also help to stabilize blood sugar levels and reduce inflammation in the body. By avoiding processed foods, sugars, and artificial additives, followers of this diet aim to minimize toxins and promote a cleaner internal environment, supporting the body's natural detoxification processes.

Moreover, the Whole Body Reset Diet promotes hydration as a cornerstone of health. Adequate water intake is emphasized throughout the cookbook, as hydration plays a vital role in cellular function, digestion, and toxin elimination.

Alongside water, herbal teas and fresh juices are encouraged as hydrating alternatives that also provide additional nutrients and antioxidants.

In addition to food choices, the diet advocates for mindful eating practices. This includes eating slowly, savoring each bite, and paying attention to hunger and satiety cues. By fostering a deeper connection with food and the eating process, individuals can cultivate a more balanced relationship with their diet and make sustainable choices that support long-term health goals.

The Whole Body Reset Diet also integrates physical activity as a complementary component to dietary changes. Regular exercise is encouraged to enhance metabolism, improve cardiovascular health, and support overall well-being. The cookbook offers guidance on incorporating exercise into daily routines, emphasizing activities that promote strength, flexibility, and cardiovascular fitness.

Furthermore, the diet emphasizes the importance of adequate sleep and stress management. Quality sleep is recognized as essential for cellular repair and hormone balance, while effective stress management techniques such as meditation, yoga, or deep breathing exercises are promoted to reduce cortisol levels and support overall mental and physical health.

Lastly, the Whole Body Reset Diet Cookbook 2024 provides practical tools and resources to support individuals on their wellness journey. This includes meal planning tips, grocery shopping lists, and a variety of delicious, nutrient-rich recipes that cater to different tastes and dietary preferences. By empowering individuals with the knowledge and tools needed to make informed choices, the cookbook aims to inspire lasting lifestyle changes that promote vitality, resilience, and overall well-being6

# Benefits of the Whole Body Reset Diet

The benefits of the Whole Body Reset Diet, as articulated through the Whole Body Reset Diet Cookbook 2024, extend far beyond mere weight management. At its core, this approach is designed to reinvigorate both body and mind, fostering a comprehensive sense of well-being that transcends fleeting dietary trends. By emphasizing whole, nutrient-dense foods, the diet aims to optimize overall health by providing a robust array of vitamins, minerals, and antioxidants essential for cellular function and vitality.

Central to the philosophy of the Whole Body Reset Diet is its focus on promoting sustainable energy levels throughout the day. By encouraging the consumption of complex carbohydrates, lean proteins, and healthy fats in balanced proportions, the diet helps stabilize blood sugar levels, preventing the energy crashes often associated with refined sugars and processed foods. This steady energy supply not only enhances daily productivity but also supports mental clarity and emotional balance.

Moreover, the Whole Body Reset Diet Cookbook 2024 champions digestive health as a cornerstone of holistic well-being. By incorporating fiber-rich fruits, vegetables, and whole grains, the diet supports optimal gut function, promoting regularity and reducing the likelihood of gastrointestinal discomfort. A healthy gut environment is crucial not only for efficient nutrient absorption but also for bolstering the immune system, thereby fortifying the body's natural defenses against illness.

Beyond physical health, this dietary approach underscores the profound impact of nutrition on mental and emotional resilience. The Whole Body Reset Diet advocates for foods rich in omega-3 fatty acids, such as salmon and walnuts, which are known to support brain health and cognitive function. Additionally, by minimizing the consumption of artificial additives and preservatives, the diet seeks to reduce inflammation throughout the body, which has been linked to a range of chronic conditions from arthritis to cardiovascular disease.

Furthermore, the Whole Body Reset Diet Cookbook 2024 promotes sustainable eating habits that can be maintained over the long term. Unlike restrictive diets that often lead to feelings of deprivation and unsustainable weight loss, this approach encourages a balanced approach to food that emphasizes enjoyment and satisfaction. By cultivating a positive relationship with food and promoting mindful eating practices, individuals are empowered to make informed choices that support their health goals without sacrificing pleasure or social connection.

In addition to its physiological benefits, the Whole Body Reset Diet places a strong emphasis on fostering a sense of community and support. The cookbook provides not only recipes but also practical tips for meal planning, grocery shopping, and preparing nutritious meals. This comprehensive guidance helps individuals navigate their dietary journey with confidence, empowering them to take ownership of their health and well-being.

Ultimately, the Whole Body Reset Diet Cookbook 2024 represents more than just a collection of recipes—it serves as a roadmap to a healthier, more vibrant life. By embracing the principles of whole-food nutrition, balanced eating, and mindful living, individuals can embark on a transformative journey towards optimal health and wellness. With each delicious and nourishing meal, they are not only nourishing their bodies but also nurturing a profound sense of vitality and vitality

# How to Use This Cookbook

To make the most of the Whole Body Reset Diet Cookbook 2024, it's essential to understand its foundational principles and how they can guide your journey to improved health and vitality. This cookbook is not just a collection of recipes but a comprehensive tool designed to help you reset and rejuvenate your body through mindful eating and balanced nutrition.

Begin by familiarizing yourself with the concept of the Whole Body Reset Diet. This approach emphasizes whole, unprocessed foods that nourish your body and support its natural detoxification processes. By focusing on nutrient-dense ingredients and minimizing refined sugars and artificial additives, you can optimize your health and energy levels.

As you explore the cookbook, take note of the guidance provided on portion sizes and meal frequency. The recipes are crafted to provide balanced meals that satisfy your hunger and fuel your body throughout the day. Whether you're planning breakfast, lunch, dinner, or snacks, each recipe is thoughtfully designed to contribute to your overall well-being.

Pay attention to the variety of recipes offered. From hearty breakfast options to satisfying dinners and nutritious snacks, the cookbook caters to different tastes and dietary preferences. Experiment with new ingredients and flavors to keep your meals exciting and enjoyable while adhering to the principles of the Whole Body Reset Diet.

Make meal planning a part of your routine. The cookbook includes sample meal plans that can guide you through a week of balanced eating. These plans are designed to help you achieve specific goals, whether it's weight loss, muscle building, or simply maintaining a healthy lifestyle. Use them as a template to customize your meals according to your individual needs and preferences.

Incorporate mindfulness into your eating habits. The Whole Body Reset Diet encourages mindful eating practices, such as paying attention to hunger and fullness cues, savoring each bite, and eating without distractions. By cultivating a mindful approach to food, you can enhance your enjoyment of meals and make healthier choices effortlessly.

Take advantage of the nutritional information provided for each recipe. The cookbook offers insights into the health benefits of key ingredients and how they contribute to your overall well-being. Use this information to make informed decisions about your food choices and to understand how each meal supports your body's nutritional needs.

Finally, view your experience with the Whole Body Reset Diet Cookbook 2024 as a journey towards holistic wellness.

Embrace the opportunity to nourish your body, mind, and spirit through delicious, nutrient-rich meals. By adopting the principles and practices outlined in the cookbook, you can cultivate lasting habits that promote vitality, energy, and a renewed sense of well-being.

# Chapter 1: Breakfast Recipes

## Superfood Smoothie Bowl

## Ingredients:

- 1 cup spinach leaves
- 1/2 cup frozen berries (such as blueberries, raspberries)
- 1/2 ripe banana
- 1/2 cup plain Greek yogurt
- 1 tbsp chia seeds
- 1/2 cup almond milk (unsweetened)
- Optional toppings: sliced almonds, coconut flakes, fresh berries

## Instructions:

1. In a blender, combine spinach, frozen berries, banana, Greek yogurt, chia seeds, and almond milk.
2. Blend until smooth and creamy.
3. Pour into a bowl and top with sliced almonds, coconut flakes, and fresh berries if desired.

# Nutritional Information:

- Calories: 320
- Protein: 18g
- Carbohydrates: 45g
- Fat: 10g
- Fiber: 12g
- Sugar: 22g

## Serving Size: 1 bowl

## Cooking Time: 5 minutes

## Ingredients:

- 1 ripe avocado
- 2 slices whole grain bread
- 2 large eggs
- Salt and pepper to taste
- Optional toppings: sliced tomatoes, microgreens, hot sauce

## Instructions:

1. Toast the whole grain bread slices until golden brown.
2. While the bread is toasting, prepare the poached eggs: Bring a small pot of water to a simmer. Crack each egg into a separate small bowl or ramekin. Gently slide the eggs into the simmering water and cook for about 3-4 minutes until the whites are set but the yolks are still runny.
3. While the eggs are poaching, mash the ripe avocado in a bowl with a fork until smooth. Season with salt and pepper to taste.
4. Spread the mashed avocado evenly onto the toasted bread slices.
5. Once the eggs are cooked, carefully remove them with a slotted spoon and place one poached egg on each avocado toast.

6. Add optional toppings if desired, such as sliced tomatoes, microgreens, or a drizzle of hot sauce.

7. Serve immediately.

## Nutritional Information (per serving):

- Calories: 320 kcal
- Protein: 14g
- Carbohydrates: 26g
- Fiber: 10g
- Total Fat: 18g
- Saturated Fat: 3g
- Cholesterol: 185mg
- Sodium: 400mg

## Serving Size: 2 slices of avocado toast with 1 poached egg each

## Cooking Time: Approximately 15 minutes

## **Ingredients**:

- Greek yogurt
- Fresh mixed berries (strawberries, blueberries, raspberries)
- Granola
- Honey or maple syrup (optional)

## **Instructions**:

1. In a serving glass or bowl, layer Greek yogurt at the bottom.
2. Add a layer of fresh mixed berries on top of the yogurt.
3. Sprinkle granola over the berries.
4. Repeat the layers until the glass or bowl is filled, ending with a layer of berries on top.
5. Drizzle with honey or maple syrup for added sweetness, if desired.

## **Nutritional Information**:  - Calories: 250

- Total Fat: 6g
- Saturated Fat: 1g
- Cholesterol: 10mg
- Sodium: 80mg

- Total Carbohydrates: 40g
- Dietary Fiber: 5g
- Sugars: 20g
- Protein: 12g

## Serving Size: 1 parfait

## Cooking Time: 5 minutes

## Ingredients:

- 1/2 cup quinoa, rinsed
- 1 cup almond milk (or any preferred milk)
- 1 tablespoon honey or maple syrup
- 1/2 teaspoon cinnamon
- 1/4 teaspoon vanilla extract
- Fresh berries and nuts for topping

## Instructions:

1. In a saucepan, combine quinoa and almond milk. Bring to a boil over medium heat.
2. Reduce heat to low, cover, and simmer for about 15 minutes, or until quinoa is tender and most of the liquid is absorbed.
3. Stir in honey or maple syrup, cinnamon, and vanilla extract.
4. Remove from heat and let it sit for 5 minutes to thicken.
5. Serve warm topped with fresh berries and nuts.

## Nutritional Information:

- Calories: 320
- Protein: 8g

- Carbohydrates: 55g
- Fiber: 5g
- Sugars: 12g
- Fat: 7g
- Saturated Fat: 1g
- Sodium: 120mg

**Serving Size**: 1 bowl

**Cooking Time**: Approximately 20 minutes

## Ingredients:

- 2 eggs
- 1/4 cup chopped bell peppers (any color)
- 1/4 cup chopped spinach
- 1/4 cup diced tomatoes
- Salt and pepper to taste
- 1 tsp olive oil
- 1 slice whole grain bread

## Instructions:

1. In a bowl, whisk together the eggs with salt and pepper.
2. Heat olive oil in a non-stick skillet over medium heat.
3. Add bell peppers, spinach, and tomatoes to the skillet. Cook until vegetables are tender, about 3-4 minutes.
4. Pour the whisked eggs over the vegetables in the skillet. Cook undisturbed until the edges set, about 2-3 minutes.
5. Carefully flip the omelette and cook for another 1-2 minutes, until eggs are fully cooked.
6. Serve hot with a slice of whole grain toast on the side.

## Nutritional Information:

- Calories: 280 kcal

- Protein: 17g
- Carbohydrates: 22g
- Fiber: 5g
- Sugar: 4g
- Fat: 14g
- Saturated Fat: 3g
- Cholesterol: 380mg
- Sodium: 480mg
- Potassium: 460mg

**Serving Size**: 1 omelette with 1 slice of toast

**Cooking Time**: Approximately 10 minutes

## Ingredients:

- 1/4 cup chia seeds
- 1 cup unsweetened almond milk
- 1 tablespoon honey or maple syrup (optional)
- Fresh berries or sliced fruits for topping

- Instructions:
  1. In a bowl, combine chia seeds and almond milk. Stir well.
  2. Add honey or maple syrup if desired for sweetness.
  3. Cover the bowl and refrigerate overnight or for at least 4 hours until thickened.
  4. Before serving, stir the pudding well to distribute the chia seeds evenly.
  5. Top with fresh berries or sliced fruits of your choice.

## Nutritional Information:

- Calories: 180
- Total Fat: 9g
- Saturated Fat: 1g
- Cholesterol: 0mg
- Sodium: 80mg
- Total Carbohydrates: 20g
- Dietary Fiber: 10g

- Sugars: 6g
- Protein: 6g

## Serving Size: 1 serving

## Cooking Time: Overnight or 4 hours refrigeration

## **Ingredients**:

- Whole wheat tortilla
- 1/2 cup cooked black beans
- 1/4 cup salsa (homemade or store-bought)
- 1/4 cup diced tomatoes
- 1/4 cup diced bell peppers
- 2 eggs, scrambled
- 1/4 cup shredded cheddar cheese
- Salt and pepper to taste
- Fresh cilantro, chopped (optional)

## **Instructions**:

1. Heat the whole wheat tortilla in a skillet over medium heat until warm.

2. In the same skillet, heat the black beans, salsa, diced tomatoes, and bell peppers until warmed through.

3. In a separate pan, scramble the eggs until fully cooked.

4. Place the warmed tortilla on a plate and layer with the scrambled eggs, black bean mixture, and shredded cheddar cheese.

5. Season with salt and pepper to taste, and garnish with chopped cilantro if desired.

6. Roll the tortilla into a burrito shape, folding in the sides as you go.

## Nutritional Information:

- Calories: 380
- Total Fat: 15g
  - Saturated Fat: 6g
  - Trans Fat: 0g
- Cholesterol: 220mg
- Sodium: 720mg
- Total Carbohydrates: 42g
  - Dietary Fiber: 10g
  - Sugars: 4g
- Protein: 20g

## Serving Size: 1 burrito

## Cooking Time: 15 minutes

# Overnight Oats with Mixed Nuts and Honey

## Ingredients:

- Rolled oats: 1/2 cup
- Greek yogurt: 1/2 cup
- Almond milk (or any milk of choice): 1/2 cup
- Mixed nuts (almonds, walnuts, pecans): 1/4 cup, chopped
- Honey: 1 tablespoon
- Fresh berries (optional): for topping

## Instructions:

1. In a mason jar or bowl, combine rolled oats, Greek yogurt, almond milk, and mixed nuts.
2. Stir well to mix all ingredients thoroughly.
3. Cover the jar or bowl and refrigerate overnight, or for at least 4 hours.
4. Before serving, drizzle honey on top and add fresh berries if desired.

## Nutritional Information:

- Calories: 350
- Protein: 15g

- Carbohydrates: 45g
- Fat: 12g
- Fiber: 7g
- Sugar: 14g
- Sodium: 100mg

**Serving Size**: 1 serving

**Cooking Time**: 10 minutes prep + overnight chilling

## **Ingredients**:

- 6 large eggs
- 1 cup chopped fresh spinach
- 1/2 cup crumbled feta cheese
- 1/4 cup diced red bell pepper
- Salt and pepper to taste
- Cooking spray or olive oil for greasing

## **Instructions**:

1. Preheat your oven to 350°F (175°C). Grease a muffin tin with cooking spray or olive oil.

2. In a mixing bowl, whisk together the eggs until well combined.

3. Stir in the chopped spinach, crumbled feta cheese, diced red bell pepper, salt, and pepper.

4. Pour the egg mixture evenly into the prepared muffin tin, filling each cup about 3/4 full.

5. Bake in the preheated oven for 20-25 minutes, or until the muffins are set and lightly golden on top.

6. Remove from the oven and allow to cool for a few minutes before serving.

## **Nutritional Information**:

- Calories: 120 kcal
- Total Fat: 8g
  - Saturated Fat: 3g
- Cholesterol: 195mg
- Sodium: 280mg
- Total Carbohydrate: 2g
  - Dietary Fiber: 0.5g
  - Sugars: 1g
- Protein: 10g

## **Serving Size**: 1 muffin

## **Cooking Time**: 20-25 minutes

## Ingredients:

- 1 ripe banana, mashed
- 2 eggs
- 1/4 cup almond flour
- 1/2 teaspoon baking powder
- Pinch of salt
- 1/2 teaspoon vanilla extract
- Coconut oil or butter for cooking
- Maple syrup for serving

## Instructions:

1. In a bowl, mash the banana until smooth.
2. Add eggs, almond flour, baking powder, salt, and vanilla extract. Mix until well combined.
3. Heat coconut oil or butter in a non-stick skillet over medium heat.
4. Pour about 1/4 cup of batter onto the skillet for each pancake.
5. Cook until bubbles form on the surface, then flip and cook until golden brown on both sides.
6. Serve warm with a drizzle of maple syrup.

## **Nutritional Information**:

- Calories: 280
- Protein: 10g
- Carbohydrates: 28g
- Fiber: 4g
- Sugars: 12g
- Fat: 15g
- Saturated Fat: 3g
- Cholesterol: 186mg
- Sodium: 360mg

## **Serving Size**: Makes about 4 pancakes

## **Cooking Time**: Approximately 15 minutes

# Chapter 2: Lunch Recipes

## Grilled Chicken Salad with Balsamic Vinaigrette

## Ingredients:

- 1 lb chicken breast, grilled and sliced
- Mixed salad greens (lettuce, spinach, arugula)
- Cherry tomatoes, halved
- Cucumber, sliced
- Red onion, thinly sliced
- Avocado, sliced
- Feta cheese, crumbled
- Balsamic vinaigrette dressing

## Instructions:

1. Grill the chicken breasts until cooked through. Let them rest, then slice thinly.
2. In a large bowl, combine the mixed salad greens, cherry tomatoes, cucumber, red onion, avocado, and feta cheese.
3. Add the sliced grilled chicken on top of the salad.

4. Drizzle with balsamic vinaigrette dressing according to taste.

5. Toss gently to combine all ingredients evenly.

6. Serve immediately and enjoy!

## Nutritional Information:

- Calories: 350 per serving
- Protein: 30g
- Carbohydrates: 15g
- Fat: 20g
- Fiber: 5g

## Serving Size: 1 salad

## Cooking Time: 20 minutes

## Ingredients:

- 1 cup quinoa, rinsed
- 2 cups water or vegetable broth
- 1 sweet potato, peeled and cubed
- 1 red bell pepper, sliced
- 1 zucchini, sliced
- 1 cup cherry tomatoes, halved
- 1 tablespoon olive oil
- Salt and pepper, to taste
- 1 avocado, sliced
- Fresh cilantro or parsley for garnish

## Instructions:

1. Preheat the oven to 400°F (200°C).
2. In a saucepan, bring the water or vegetable broth to a boil. Add the quinoa, reduce heat to low, cover, and simmer for about 15-20 minutes or until quinoa is cooked and water is absorbed.
3. Meanwhile, toss the sweet potato, red bell pepper, zucchini, and cherry tomatoes with olive oil, salt, and pepper on a baking sheet.

4. Roast the vegetables in the preheated oven for 20-25 minutes, or until they are tender and lightly browned.

5. To assemble the Buddha bowls, divide the cooked quinoa among serving bowls.

6. Top each bowl with roasted vegetables and avocado slices.

7. Garnish with fresh cilantro or parsley.

8. Serve warm and enjoy!

## Nutritional Information:

- Calories: 350
- Total Fat: 15g
- Saturated Fat: 2g
- Cholesterol: 0mg
- Sodium: 200mg
- Total Carbohydrate: 48g
- Dietary Fiber: 10g
- Total Sugars: 6g
- Protein: 10g

## Serving Size: 1 bowl

## Cooking Time: 45 minutes (including preparation and roasting)

## Ingredients:

- Whole grain tortilla
- Sliced turkey breast
- Ripe avocado, sliced
- Mixed greens (such as spinach or arugula)
- Tomato, thinly sliced
- Red onion, thinly sliced
- Hummus or Greek yogurt spread
- Optional: Sliced cucumber, bell peppers, or other vegetables of choice

## Instructions:

1. Lay the whole grain tortilla flat on a clean surface.
2. Spread a generous layer of hummus or Greek yogurt spread over the tortilla.
3. Layer the sliced turkey breast evenly over the spread.
4. Arrange slices of avocado, tomato, red onion, and any additional vegetables over the turkey.
5. Add a handful of mixed greens on top of the vegetables.
6. Carefully fold the sides of the tortilla towards the center, then roll it tightly from bottom to top to create a wrap.

7. Secure with toothpicks if necessary, then slice in half diagonally.

## Nutritional Information:

- Calories per serving: Approximately 350 kcal
- Protein: 25g
- Carbohydrates: 30g
- Fiber: 8g
- Total Fat: 15g
- Saturated Fat: 3g
- Sodium: 450mg

## Serving Size: 1 wrap

## Cooking Time: 15 minutes

## **Ingredients:**

- 1 cup dried green or brown lentils, rinsed
- 1 onion, finely chopped
- 2 carrots, diced
- 2 celery stalks, diced
- 3 garlic cloves, minced
- 1 tablespoon olive oil
- 1 teaspoon dried thyme
- 1 teaspoon dried oregano
- 1 bay leaf
- 6 cups vegetable broth
- Salt and pepper to taste
- Fresh parsley or cilantro, chopped (for garnish)

## **Instructions:**

1. In a large pot, heat olive oil over medium heat. Add chopped onion, carrots, and celery. Sauté for 5-7 minutes until vegetables are softened.

2. Add minced garlic, dried thyme, dried oregano, and bay leaf. Cook for another 1-2 minutes until fragrant.

3. Stir in rinsed lentils and vegetable broth. Bring to a boil, then reduce heat to low. Cover and simmer for 25-30 minutes, or until lentils are tender.

4. Season with salt and pepper to taste. Remove bay leaf.

5. Serve hot, garnished with chopped fresh parsley or cilantro.

## Nutritional Information:

- Calories: 250 per serving
- Total Fat: 4g
- Sodium: 800mg
- Total Carbohydrates: 40g
- Dietary Fiber: 15g
- Protein: 15g

## Serving Size: 1 cup

## Cooking Time: 40 minutes

# Caprese Salad with Fresh Mozzarella and Basil

## Ingredients:

- Fresh mozzarella cheese, sliced
- Fresh tomatoes, sliced
- Fresh basil leaves
- Extra virgin olive oil
- Balsamic vinegar
- Salt and pepper to taste

## Instructions:

1. Arrange slices of fresh mozzarella and tomatoes on a serving plate.
2. Tuck fresh basil leaves between the cheese and tomatoes.
3. Drizzle with extra virgin olive oil and balsamic vinegar.
4. Season with salt and pepper to taste.
5. Serve immediately and enjoy the refreshing flavors.

## Nutritional Information:

- Calories: 250 kcal
- Carbohydrates: 5g

- Protein: 12g
- Fat: 20g
- Fiber: 1g

## Serving Size: 1 serving

## Cooking Time: 10 minutes

## **Ingredients**:

- 2 medium sweet potatoes
- 1 can (15 ounces) chickpeas, drained and rinsed
- 2 cups fresh spinach, chopped
- 1/2 red bell pepper, diced
- 1/4 cup red onion, finely chopped
- 1 clove garlic, minced
- 1 tablespoon olive oil
- 1 teaspoon ground cumin
- 1/2 teaspoon smoked paprika
- Salt and pepper to taste
- Optional toppings: Greek yogurt, chopped cilantro, lime wedges

## **Instructions**:

1. Preheat the oven to 400°F (200°C).
2. Scrub the sweet potatoes and pierce them several times with a fork. Place them on a baking sheet lined with parchment paper and bake for 45-60 minutes, or until tender.

3. In a large skillet, heat olive oil over medium heat. Add red onion and bell pepper, sautéing until softened, about 5 minutes.

4. Add garlic, cumin, smoked paprika, salt, and pepper. Cook for another 1-2 minutes until fragrant.

5. Stir in chickpeas and spinach. Cook until spinach is wilted and chickpeas are heated through, about 3-4 minutes.

6. Once sweet potatoes are cooked, slice them open and fluff the flesh with a fork.

7. Divide the chickpea and spinach mixture evenly among the sweet potatoes.

8. Garnish with optional toppings such as Greek yogurt, chopped cilantro, and a squeeze of fresh lime juice.

## Nutritional Information:

- Calories: 320 kcal
- Protein: 10g
- Carbohydrates: 55g
- Fat: 8g
- Fiber: 10g

## Serving Size: 1 stuffed sweet potato

## Cooking Time: 60 minutes

## **Ingredients**:

- 1 can (5 oz) of tuna, drained
- 1/4 cup Greek yogurt
- 1 tablespoon lemon juice
- 1/4 teaspoon garlic powder
- 1/4 teaspoon onion powder
- Salt and pepper to taste
- 2 cups mixed greens
- 1/2 cucumber, sliced
- 1/2 cup cherry tomatoes, halved
- 1/4 red onion, thinly sliced
- Optional: 1 tablespoon chopped fresh herbs (such as parsley or dill)

## **Instructions**:

1. In a small bowl, mix together the Greek yogurt, lemon juice, garlic powder, onion powder, salt, and pepper until well combined.
2. In a larger bowl, combine the drained tuna with the Greek yogurt dressing, stirring gently to coat the tuna evenly.
3. Arrange the mixed greens, cucumber slices, cherry tomatoes, and red onion on a plate or in a bowl.
4. Top the salad with the tuna mixture.

5. Optional: Garnish with chopped fresh herbs if desired.

6. Serve immediately and enjoy!

## Nutritional Information:

- Calories: 250 kcal
- Protein: 30g
- Carbohydrates: 10g
- Fat: 10g
- Fiber: 3g
- Sodium: 350mg

## Serving Size: 1 serving

## Cooking Time: 15 minutes

# Grilled Veggie Sandwich with Pesto Spread

## Ingredients:

- Whole grain bread slices
- Zucchini, sliced lengthwise
- Bell peppers (red, yellow, or orange), sliced
- Eggplant, sliced
- Red onion, thinly sliced
- Pesto sauce (homemade or store-bought)
- Olive oil
- Salt and pepper to taste

## Instructions:

1. Preheat a grill pan or outdoor grill over medium heat.
2. Brush the sliced zucchini, bell peppers, eggplant, and red onion with olive oil. Season with salt and pepper.
3. Grill the vegetables until tender and slightly charred, about 3-4 minutes per side.
4. While grilling, lightly toast the whole grain bread slices.
5. Spread pesto sauce generously on one side of each toasted bread slice.
6. Arrange the grilled vegetables on top of the pesto spread on one bread slice.

7. Place the other bread slice on top to form a sandwich.

8. Optionally, press the sandwich lightly and cut it in half.

## Nutritional Information:

- Calories per serving: Approximately 300 kcal
- Total Fat: 12g
- Saturated Fat: 2g
- Cholesterol: 0mg
- Sodium: 450mg
- Total Carbohydrates: 40g
- Dietary Fiber: 8g
- Sugars: 8g
- Protein: 10g

## Serving Size: 1 sandwich

## Cooking Time: Approximately 15 minutes

## **Ingredients**:

- Romaine lettuce, chopped
- Grilled chicken breast, sliced
- Parmesan cheese, grated
- Whole wheat croutons
- Caesar dressing (homemade or store-bought)

## **Instructions**:

1. In a large bowl, combine chopped romaine lettuce with grilled chicken breast slices.
2. Sprinkle grated Parmesan cheese and whole wheat croutons over the salad.
3. Drizzle Caesar dressing generously over the salad mixture.
4. Toss gently to coat all ingredients evenly.
5. Serve immediately, optionally garnished with additional Parmesan cheese and cracked black pepper.

## **Nutritional Information**:

- Calories: 350 kcal
- Protein: 30g
- Carbohydrates: 15g
- Fat: 20g

- Fiber: 5g

**Serving Size**: 1 serving

**Cooking Time**: 20 minutes

# Whole Wheat Pasta Primavera

## **Ingredients:**

- 8 oz whole wheat pasta
- 1 tbsp olive oil
- 2 cloves garlic, minced
- 1 small onion, thinly sliced
- 1 red bell pepper, thinly sliced
- 1 yellow bell pepper, thinly sliced
- 1 zucchini, halved and thinly sliced
- 1 cup cherry tomatoes, halved
- 1/2 cup vegetable broth
- Salt and pepper to taste
- 1/4 cup grated Parmesan cheese (optional)
- Fresh basil leaves, chopped (for garnish)

## **Instructions:**

1. Cook the whole wheat pasta according to package instructions until al dente. Drain and set aside.

2. In a large skillet, heat olive oil over medium heat. Add garlic and onion, sauté until fragrant and onion is translucent.

3. Add bell peppers, zucchini, and cherry tomatoes to the skillet. Cook, stirring occasionally, until vegetables are tender-crisp.

4. Pour vegetable broth into the skillet and bring to a simmer. Season with salt and pepper to taste.

5. Add cooked pasta to the skillet, tossing gently to combine with the vegetables and broth.

6. Remove from heat and sprinkle with Parmesan cheese, if using. Garnish with chopped basil leaves.

## Nutritional Information:

- Calories: 350
- Protein: 12g
- Carbohydrates: 55g
- Fat: 10g
- Fiber: 8g
- Sugar: 6g
- Sodium: 350mg

## Serving Size: 1 serving

## Cooking Time: 20 minutes

# Chapter 3: Dinner Recipes

## Baked Salmon with Asparagus

## Ingredients:

- 4 salmon fillets (6 oz each)
- 1 bunch of asparagus, trimmed
- 2 tablespoons olive oil
- 2 cloves garlic, minced
- 1 lemon, sliced
- Salt and pepper to taste

## Instructions:

1. Preheat the oven to 400°F (200°C). Line a baking sheet with parchment paper.

2. Place the salmon fillets on the prepared baking sheet. Arrange the asparagus around the salmon.

3. Drizzle olive oil over the salmon and asparagus. Season with minced garlic, salt, and pepper.

4. Place lemon slices on top of each salmon fillet.

5. Bake in the preheated oven for 12-15 minutes, or until the salmon is cooked through and flakes easily with a fork.

6. Remove from the oven and serve immediately.

## Nutritional Information:

- Calories: 350
- Protein: 34g
- Carbohydrates: 6g
- Fat: 20g
- Fiber: 3g
- Sugar: 2g
- Sodium: 300mg

## Serving Size: 1 salmon fillet with asparagus

## Cooking Time: 15 minutes

## **Ingredients**:

- 4 large bell peppers, any color
- 1 cup quinoa, rinsed
- 1 ½ cups vegetable broth
- 1 can (15 oz) black beans, drained and rinsed
- 1 cup corn kernels (fresh or frozen)
- 1 cup diced tomatoes
- 1 teaspoon cumin
- 1 teaspoon chili powder
- Salt and pepper, to taste
- ½ cup shredded cheddar cheese (optional)
- Fresh cilantro, chopped (for garnish)

## **Instructions**:

1. Preheat oven to 375°F (190°C). Cut the tops off the bell peppers and remove the seeds and membranes.

2. In a medium saucepan, bring the vegetable broth to a boil. Add quinoa, reduce heat to low, cover, and simmer for 15-20 minutes, or until quinoa is cooked and liquid is absorbed.

3. In a large mixing bowl, combine cooked quinoa, black beans, corn, diced tomatoes, cumin, chili powder, salt, and pepper. Mix well.

4. Stuff each bell pepper with the quinoa mixture and place them in a baking dish. If using cheese, sprinkle it over the stuffed peppers.

5. Cover the dish with foil and bake for 25-30 minutes, or until the peppers are tender.

6. Remove foil and bake for an additional 5-10 minutes, or until cheese is melted and bubbly (if using).

7. Remove from oven and let cool slightly before serving. Garnish with chopped cilantro if desired.

## Nutritional Information:

- Calories: 320 per serving
- Total Fat: 6g
  - Saturated Fat: 2.5g
  - Trans Fat: 0g
- Cholesterol: 10mg
- Sodium: 480mg
- Total Carbohydrates: 55g
  - Dietary Fiber: 12g
  - Sugars: 8g
- Protein: 14g

## Serving Size: 1 stuffed bell pepper

## Cooking Time: 45-50 minutes

## **Ingredients**:

- 4 sirloin steaks, about 6 oz each
- 4 tablespoons unsalted butter, softened
- 4 cloves garlic, minced
- Salt and pepper to taste
- Fresh parsley, chopped (for garnish)

## **Instructions**:

1. Preheat grill to medium-high heat.
2. In a small bowl, combine softened butter, minced garlic, salt, and pepper.
3. Generously season both sides of the steaks with salt and pepper.
4. Grill steaks for about 4-5 minutes per side, or until desired doneness (about 145°F for medium-rare).
5. Remove steaks from grill and let rest for 5 minutes.
6. Top each steak with a tablespoon of garlic butter mixture and garnish with chopped parsley before serving.

## **Nutritional Information**:

- Calories: 450
- Protein: 40g

- Carbohydrates: 1g
- Fat: 32g
- Fiber: 0g
- Sugar: 0g
- Sodium: 350mg

## Serving Size: 1 steak with garlic butter

## Cooking Time: 20 minutes

## Ingredients:

- 1 block extra-firm tofu, pressed and cubed
- 2 tablespoons soy sauce
- 1 tablespoon sesame oil
- 1 tablespoon cornstarch
- 1 tablespoon vegetable oil
- 1 onion, sliced
- 2 cloves garlic, minced
- 1 bell pepper, thinly sliced
- 1 cup broccoli florets
- 1 cup sliced mushrooms
- Salt and pepper, to taste
- Cooked brown rice or quinoa, for serving

## Instructions:

1. In a bowl, toss cubed tofu with soy sauce, sesame oil, and cornstarch until coated.

2. Heat vegetable oil in a large skillet or wok over medium-high heat. Add tofu cubes and cook until golden and crispy on all sides, about 5-7 minutes. Remove tofu from skillet and set aside.

3. In the same skillet, add onion and garlic. Sauté until fragrant, about 2 minutes.

4. Add bell pepper, broccoli, and mushrooms. Stir-fry for 5-7 minutes until vegetables are tender-crisp.

5. Return tofu to the skillet. Season with salt and pepper to taste. Stir well to combine.

6. Serve hot over cooked brown rice or quinoa.

## Nutritional Information:

- Calories: 320 kcal
- Protein: 18g
- Carbohydrates: 25g
- Fiber: 6g
- Sugar: 5g
- Fat: 18g
- Saturated Fat: 3g
- Sodium: 720mg
- Cholesterol: 0mg

## Serving Size: 1 serving

## Cooking Time: 25 minutes

# Ingredients:

- 1 lb boneless, skinless chicken breast, cut into chunks
- 1 red bell pepper, cut into chunks
- 1 yellow bell pepper, cut into chunks
- 1 red onion, cut into chunks
- Zest and juice of 1 lemon
- 2 cloves garlic, minced
- 2 tbsp olive oil
- Salt and pepper, to taste
- Wooden or metal skewers

# Instructions:

1. In a bowl, combine lemon zest, lemon juice, minced garlic, olive oil, salt, and pepper.

2. Add chicken chunks to the marinade, ensuring they are evenly coated. Marinate in the refrigerator for at least 30 minutes.

3. Preheat grill or grill pan over medium-high heat.

4. Thread marinated chicken, bell peppers, and onion onto skewers, alternating ingredients.

5. Grill kebabs for 8-10 minutes, turning occasionally, until chicken is cooked through and vegetables are tender.

6. Serve hot, garnished with fresh herbs if desired.

## Nutritional Information:

- Calories: 280 kcal
- Protein: 30g
- Carbohydrates: 10g
- Fiber: 2g
- Sugars: 4g
- Fat: 13g
- Saturated Fat: 2g
- Cholesterol: 80mg
- Sodium: 300mg

## Serving Size: 1 kebab (serves 2-3)

## Cooking Time: 20 minutes

## **Ingredients**:

- 1 lb shrimp, peeled and deveined
- 4 medium zucchini, spiralized into noodles
- 1 cup cherry tomatoes, halved
- 1/4 cup pesto sauce
- 2 cloves garlic, minced
- Salt and pepper to taste
- Olive oil for cooking

## **Instructions**:

1. Heat olive oil in a large skillet over medium heat. Add minced garlic and sauté until fragrant.
2. Add shrimp to the skillet and cook until pink and opaque, about 2-3 minutes per side. Season with salt and pepper.
3. Stir in cherry tomatoes and cook for another 1-2 minutes until tomatoes start to soften.
4. Add zucchini noodles to the skillet and toss with the shrimp and tomatoes.
5. Cook for 2-3 minutes, stirring occasionally, until zucchini noodles are just tender.
6. Remove skillet from heat and stir in pesto sauce until everything is well coated.

## Nutritional Information:

- Calories: 320
- Protein: 30g
- Carbohydrates: 10g
- Fat: 18g
- Fiber: 3g
- Sugar: 6g

## Serving Size: 4 servings

## Cooking Time: 20 minutes

# Stuffed Portobello Mushrooms with Quinoa and Spinach

## Ingredients:

- 4 large Portobello mushrooms
- 1 cup quinoa, cooked
- 2 cups fresh spinach, chopped
- 1/2 cup cherry tomatoes, diced
- 1/4 cup red onion, finely chopped
- 2 cloves garlic, minced
- 1/2 cup feta cheese, crumbled
- Salt and pepper to taste
- Olive oil for drizzling

## Instructions:

1. Preheat oven to 375°F (190°C). Line a baking sheet with parchment paper.

2. Clean the Portobello mushrooms and remove the stems. Place them on the baking sheet, gill side up.

3. In a skillet, heat olive oil over medium heat. Add minced garlic and chopped red onion, sauté until fragrant.

4. Add chopped spinach to the skillet and cook until wilted.

5. In a bowl, combine cooked quinoa, sautéed vegetables, diced cherry tomatoes, and crumbled feta cheese. Season with salt and pepper.

6. Spoon the quinoa mixture into each Portobello mushroom cap, pressing gently to pack it in.

7. Drizzle olive oil over the stuffed mushrooms and bake in the preheated oven for 20-25 minutes, or until the mushrooms are tender and the filling is heated through.

8. Remove from the oven and let cool slightly before serving.

## Nutritional Information:

- Calories: 280
- Total Fat: 12g
  - Saturated Fat: 4g
- Cholesterol: 15mg
- Sodium: 350mg
- Total Carbohydrates: 32g
  - Dietary Fiber: 6g
  - Sugars: 4g
- Protein: 12g

## Serving Size: 1 stuffed Portobello mushroom

## Cooking Time: 40 minutes

## **Ingredients**:

- 4 bone-in, skin-on chicken thighs
- 2 tablespoons olive oil
- 2 cloves garlic, minced
- 1 lemon, zested and juiced
- 1 teaspoon dried thyme
- 1 teaspoon dried rosemary
- Salt and pepper to taste

## **Instructions**:

1. Preheat oven to 400°F (200°C). Line a baking sheet with parchment paper.
2. In a small bowl, combine olive oil, minced garlic, lemon zest, lemon juice, thyme, rosemary, salt, and pepper.
3. Place chicken thighs on the prepared baking sheet. Brush both sides with the herb mixture.
4. Roast in the preheated oven for 30-35 minutes, or until chicken is cooked through and skin is crispy.
5. Remove from oven and let rest for 5 minutes before serving.

## **Nutritional Information**:

- Calories: 320
- Total Fat: 21g
- Saturated Fat: 5g
- Cholesterol: 140mg
- Sodium: 360mg
- Carbohydrates: 2g
- Fiber: 0g
- Sugars: 0g
- Protein: 30g

**Serving Size**: 1 chicken thigh

**Cooking Time**: 30-35 minutes

# Cauliflower Rice Stir-Fry with Shrimp

## Ingredients:

- 1 lb shrimp, peeled and deveined
- 1 head cauliflower, grated into rice-sized pieces
- 1 red bell pepper, sliced
- 1 cup snap peas
- 2 cloves garlic, minced
- 1 tbsp ginger, minced
- 2 tbsp low-sodium soy sauce
- 1 tbsp sesame oil
- Salt and pepper to taste
- Fresh cilantro for garnish

## Instructions:

1. Heat sesame oil in a large skillet over medium-high heat.
2. Add garlic and ginger, sauté for 1 minute until fragrant.
3. Add shrimp to the skillet and cook until pink and opaque, about 3-4 minutes. Remove shrimp and set aside.
4. In the same skillet, add cauliflower rice, bell pepper, and snap peas. Cook for 5-6 minutes until vegetables are tender.
5. Return shrimp to the skillet. Stir in soy sauce, and season with salt and pepper to taste. Cook for an additional 2 minutes to heat through.
6. Serve hot, garnished with fresh cilantro.

## Nutritional Information:

- Calories: 250 per serving
- Protein: 30g
- Carbohydrates: 15g
- Fat: 8g
- Fiber: 5g

## Serving Size: 4 servings

## Cooking Time: 20 minutes

# Baked Cod with Tomato and Olive Relish

## Ingredients:

- 4 cod fillets (6 ounces each)
- 1 cup cherry tomatoes, halved
- 1/2 cup Kalamata olives, pitted and chopped
- 2 tablespoons extra virgin olive oil
- 2 cloves garlic, minced
- 1 tablespoon capers, drained
- 1 tablespoon fresh lemon juice
- Salt and pepper to taste
- Fresh parsley, chopped (for garnish)

## Instructions:

1. Preheat the oven to 400°F (200°C). Line a baking sheet with parchment paper.

2. In a small bowl, combine the cherry tomatoes, olives, olive oil, garlic, capers, lemon juice, salt, and pepper. Mix well to make the relish.

3. Place the cod fillets on the prepared baking sheet. Season them with salt and pepper.

4. Spoon the tomato and olive relish evenly over each cod fillet.

5. Bake in the preheated oven for 15-20 minutes, or until the cod is opaque and flakes easily with a fork.

6. Remove from the oven and garnish with fresh chopped parsley before serving.

## Nutritional Information:

- Calories: 280
- Total Fat: 14g
- Saturated Fat: 2g
- Cholesterol: 70mg
- Sodium: 480mg
- Total Carbohydrates: 5g
- Dietary Fiber: 2g
- Sugars: 2g
- Protein: 32g

## Serving Size: 1 cod fillet with relish

## Cooking Time: 20 minutes

# Chapter 4: Dessert Recipes

## Apple Slices with Almond Butter

## Ingredients:

- 1 apple, sliced
- 2 tablespoons almond butter


- Instructions:
  1. Wash and core the apple, then slice it into thin rounds or wedges.
  2. Spread almond butter evenly on each apple slice.

## Nutritional Information:

- Calories per serving: 160
- Total Fat: 9g
- Saturated Fat: 1g
- Trans Fat: 0g
- Cholesterol: 0mg
- Sodium: 5mg
- Total Carbohydrates: 18g

- Dietary Fiber: 4g
- Sugars: 12g
- Protein: 4g

## Serving Size: 1 serving

## Cooking Time: None

## Ingredients:

- 1 cup mixed nuts (almonds, walnuts, cashews)
- 1/2 cup dried cranberries
- 1/2 cup dried apricots, chopped
- 1/4 cup pumpkin seeds
- 1/4 cup dark chocolate chips (optional)

## Instructions:

1. In a large mixing bowl, combine all the ingredients: mixed nuts, dried cranberries, chopped dried apricots, pumpkin seeds, and dark chocolate chips if using.
2. Toss gently to mix evenly.
3. Store in an airtight container for up to two weeks.

## Nutritional Information:

- Calories: 180
- Total Fat: 11g
  - Saturated Fat: 2g
  - Trans Fat: 0g
- Cholesterol: 0mg
- Sodium: 5mg
- Total Carbohydrates: 19g

   - Dietary Fiber: 3g
   - Sugars: 13g
 - Protein: 4g

## Serving Size: 1/4 cup

## Cooking Time: None

## Ingredients:

- Greek yogurt (unsweetened)
- Fresh berries (e.g., strawberries, blueberries, raspberries)
- Honey (optional, for drizzling)

## Instructions:

1. Spoon Greek yogurt into a bowl or serving dish.
2. Wash and prepare fresh berries, then arrange them on top of the yogurt.
3. Drizzle with honey, if desired, for added sweetness.
4. Serve immediately and enjoy!

## Nutritional Information:

- Calories per serving: 150
- Total Fat: 3g
- Cholesterol: 10mg
- Sodium: 50mg
- Total Carbohydrates: 20g
- Dietary Fiber: 2g
- Sugars: 16g

- Protein: 10g

**Serving Size**: 1 bowl

**Cooking Time**: None

# Hummus and Veggie Sticks

## Ingredients:

- 1 cup chickpeas, drained and rinsed
- 2 tablespoons tahini
- 2 tablespoons lemon juice
- 1 garlic clove, minced
- 2 tablespoons olive oil
- Salt and pepper to taste
- Assorted vegetable sticks (carrots, cucumber, bell peppers) for serving

## Instructions:

1. In a food processor, combine chickpeas, tahini, lemon juice, garlic, olive oil, salt, and pepper.
2. Blend until smooth and creamy, adding water as needed to achieve desired consistency.
3. Transfer hummus to a serving bowl and drizzle with a little extra olive oil if desired.
4. Serve with assorted vegetable sticks for dipping.

## Nutritional Information:

- Calories: 150
- Total Fat: 9g

- Saturated Fat: 1g
- Sodium: 150mg
- Carbohydrates: 14g
- Fiber: 4g
- Sugars: 2g
- Protein: 5g

**Serving Size**: Makes about 1 cup of hummus, serving approximately 4 people as an appetizer.

**Cooking Time**: Prep Time: 10 minutes; Total Time: 10 minutes.

## **Ingredients**:

- Fresh strawberries
- Dark chocolate (at least 70% cocoa)

## **Instructions**:

1. Wash and dry the strawberries thoroughly.
2. Melt the dark chocolate in a heatproof bowl over a pot of simmering water, stirring until smooth.
3. Dip each strawberry into the melted chocolate, coating it evenly.
4. Place the coated strawberries on a parchment-lined baking sheet.
5. Refrigerate for about 15-20 minutes, or until the chocolate hardens.
6. Serve and enjoy!

## **Nutritional Information**:

- Calories: Approximately 60 kcal
- Protein: 1g
- Fat: 3g
- Carbohydrates: 7g
- Fiber: 2g

- Sugar: 4g
- Sodium: 0mg

**Serving Size**: 4-6 strawberries

**Cooking Time**: 30 minutes

# Conclusion

The conclusion of the Whole Body Reset Diet Cookbook 2024 serves as a culmination of the journey towards holistic wellness and vitality. It encapsulates the core principles and benefits of adopting the Whole Body Reset Diet as a lifestyle choice rather than a temporary regimen. Throughout the cookbook, the emphasis has been on nourishing the body with nutrient-dense foods, supporting its natural detoxification processes, and promoting overall health.

In this final section, readers are encouraged to reflect on their experience with the cookbook and the positive changes they have observed in their health and well-being. It reinforces the idea that healthy eating is not about deprivation but about making informed choices that support long-term health goals. By embracing the recipes and meal plans provided, individuals can sustainably manage their weight, increase energy levels, and enhance their overall quality of life.

The conclusion also provides practical tips and encouragement for maintaining the momentum gained from using the cookbook. It emphasizes the importance of consistency, mindfulness in eating habits, and adapting recipes to personal preferences and dietary needs. Readers are empowered to continue exploring new flavors, ingredients, and cooking techniques that align with the principles of the Whole Body Reset Diet.

Moreover, the conclusion may include testimonials or success stories from individuals who have benefited from following the Whole Body Reset Diet. These personal accounts serve to inspire and motivate readers, showcasing real-life examples of how the cookbook's recipes and principles can positively impact health outcomes.

Lastly, the conclusion may offer guidance on transitioning beyond the cookbook, encouraging readers to integrate the principles learned into their daily lives. This might involve creating personalized meal plans, practicing mindful eating, and seeking ongoing support from health professionals or community resources.

Ultimately, the conclusion of the Whole Body Reset Diet Cookbook 2024 reinforces the idea that achieving and maintaining optimal health is a journey, and this cookbook serves as a valuable companion along the way—a testament to the power of nutritious eating in enhancing both physical vitality and overall well-being.